How To Be Good At Sex

How To Push Your Partners Buttons, How To Have A Crazy Sex Life And How To Be Good At Sex Every Time!

Table of Contents

Do You Want More Books?

How would you like books arriving in your inbox each week?

Don't worry they are FREE!

We publish books on all sorts of non-fiction niches and send them out to our subscribers each week to spread the love.

All you have to do is sign up and you're good to go!

Just go to the link at the end of this book, sign up, sit back and wait for your book downloads to arrive!

We couldn't have made it any easier! Enjoy!

Introduction

I want to thank you and congratulate you for purchasing the book, "How To Be Good At Sex, *How To Push Your Partners Buttons, How To Have A Crazy Sex Life And How To Be Good At Sex Every Time!*"

This book contains proven steps and strategies on how to get the spice back in your cold and virtually nonexistent sex life.

When it comes to sex, men are like instant noodles, ready to serve and eat. Women on the other hand, are similar to a three-course meal that requires meticulous planning on preparation much before hand and served at intervals while dining.

Though this is a well-known phenomenon, men and women still feel frustrated when they do not share a mutual understanding on the subject of pleasuring each other. Read along and uncover answers to your most private questions.

Thanks again for purchasing this book, I hope you enjoy it!

Chapter 1: Improving Your Sex Life

Let's be realistic and accept the fact that good sex happens to those willing to explore their bodies and the bodies of their partners. Sex is a very intimate experience between two people; especially when you engage in sex within relationships.

There are many factors that control your sex life; erratic working hours, work pressures, children, living with extended family, economic obligations, health, hormonal changes with age, and most importantly compatibility.

Men and women lead busy lives and are often devoid of imagination and the unwillingness to experiment due to stress and fatigue. Engaging in good sex does not require extra ordinary skills or tools; little change and doing things different can lead to a gratifying experience. This requires effort and isn't difficult to achieve.

Recharge your sexual batteries by doing things that allow you to break free from your hectic schedules. When you're relaxed and feeling good about yourself, sex will begin to seem within the realm of possibility all over again.

During the early years of courtship, sex is almost transcendental. It is spontaneous, thrilling, and frequent. This takes place because as humans we are curious creatures, and anything that is unexplored or unachieved grabs our interest; naturally we enthusiastically go the extra mile to achieve it.

The smell, the touch and the taste of the person you are deeply in love with engages you in passionate lovemaking causing momentary amnesia while you act on your instincts.

As months and years pass by, a couple's sex life takes a nosedive; it is taken for granted that you could have sex with this particular person in the comforts of your own home whenever you please. Now that the chase is over, and your lives are scheduled as well as organized in a defined pattern, there remains nothing rousing about sex any more, and couples spends weeks and even months without even indulging in foreplay.

Eventually partners make no efforts to impress each other and the 'comfort levels' (though healthy in any relationship), more often than not is destructive for leading healthy sex lives. Couples discontinue dressing up and grooming themselves for their partners.

Men no longer send flowers to their wives and women stop acting like girlfriends after they are married. Has it ever occurred to you, why are men more attracted to their girlfriends than they are to their wives even though they may marry the same person they dated?

This 'role playing' by both genders certainly hampers sex lives to some degree as times goes by.

Understanding Men

Everyone knows men love watching pornography, and I personally have no problems if my partner wishes to watch erotic naked bodies. As women, we need to be open enough to understand that men are 'visual creatures', and if they find bare bodies of women on a screen or in magazines arousing, it does not harm your relationship and nor does it question his loyalty towards you.

I certainly do not imply that your husband or boyfriend expects you to behave like a porn star against your will.

Some men are juvenile when it comes to setting boundaries in bed. Though many adolescent males, thanks to their raging hormone levels and many men as well who have not entirely snapped out of boyhood, demand unreasonable favours from the women they sleep with.

A percentage of married men as well, behave poorly and express the desire to experiment with a certain position they find arousing which their partners may not find desirable. It takes maturity, healthy communication along with a deep understanding of each other's needs.

Men need to assure women that there is nothing to be anxious about, a mentally relaxed woman is turned on faster than one that is full of anxiety.

A study at the University of Virginia found that the foremost predictor of a woman's marital happiness was the level of her husband's emotional engagement. If couples spend quality time together, they're happier. When they feeling disconnected, their relationship and sex life suffers.

Women need to feel close to their man to be motivated to make love, and men often need sex to feel close to their women. Make the first move --do something simple like thanking your husband for taking out the trash or paying the bills on time.

When you show a little gratitude, it's a huge bonding moment for men. In response, men start tuning into their wife's needs.

What Men Want

Men are very attracted to inhibited women; they desire to be with someone who is enthusiastic as a lover. They feel better about themselves when women express they're looking forward to doing things with them. Sexual desires are like an appetite, everyone wants to try different flavors. Men want someone willing to explore feelings and new sensations.

When a woman genuinely complements the man in her life, she never lacks his affection. Men generally don't follow instructions -- but in bed, they love it when women tell them what to do.

All men have fantasies and they will share them with their partners if she seems interested to know and act on them.

It's healthy to discuss sexual desires and negotiate on how both partners like to be touched.

Men reciprocate to someone who initiates sex. So, don't always expect a man to make the first move. Some men love dirty talk – The order in which their attention follows, is that they always notice with their eyes, listen to hints that make them feel wanted, and then, be aware of their feelings; that's how they're wired. Talking dirty arouses a man and his imagination wanders, this turns them on psychologically.

Sex is all about touch. Paying attention on how to precisely use touch does wonders for both men and women. Men may not necessarily like to be soft, loving, and romantic after the initial period; they like to be a little rough.

If a woman turns into being a brat in the bedroom it makes a man beg for more. The biggest turn on for a guy is when he knows that he pleased you.

Understanding Women

Women are emotional creatures; they are wired differently than men. An emotionally happy woman will delight a man like a king in bed. Pleasuring comes naturally to her when she is eager to experience an intimate moment with her partner.

Men must be willing to acknowledge a woman's emotional and physical needs if they want their partners to be willing to experiment. By no means has this meant using manipulation or deceit. Women have a natural gift of the sixth sense and are very intuitive at recognizing fact from fiction.

Women crave to be understood and taken care of, when they are genuinely happy in a relationship; they feel like a woman in the true sense and are willing to explore their bodies and the bodies of their partners without inhibitions.

Many women suffer from a poor body image due to the unrealistic trends the fashion industry psychologically imposes. Women admit that while they lie naked in bed with their partners, they constantly worry about how they appear and shy away from engaging in new things.

In reality, men do not fuss over how their partners appear when nude. Remember, if he feels you're unattractive, he wouldn't be in bed with you in the first place.

Every woman is different, and several don't even orgasm with the same guy for the first couple of times they make love. A woman has to feel comfortable, and men have to figure out what ticks her sexually. Some women enjoy wet, sloppy kisses, breast stimulation while others just hate it, some might be averse to being on top or going down on men, while some love it.

Ever wondered why a woman, who once was sexual, now seems numb and frigid. There could be many reasons to this, child birth, stress, depression, being aware and enduring a cheating partner, prolonged use of contraceptives or other medication, ailments and illnesses, hormonal changes. Understanding a woman's needs and allowing her the time to open up is a gentleman's prerogative.

What Women Want

Women are emotionally sensitive creatures who feel everything, and the same goes with sex. Unlike men, women take time to be turned on. Expecting your partner to jump into bed with you just because you're in the mood isn't fair. Express your desire in a way that doesn't make her feel obligated.

Indulging in foreplay is always better before getting your act together. Understand what turns her on; a woman's body yearns to be explored, she may not always admit to it, but she secretly desires her partner to do things that please her sexually.

Some women also like dirty sex but may not necessarily mention it for the fear of being judged, especially if they have been brought up in an orthodox environment or have rigged religious beliefs.

Research at the University of Washington reveals that women are much more likely to be satisfied with their relationship and ask for more sex when men pitch in around the house, just helping around by wiping the counter, unloading the dishwasher can be very helpful in building up mutual respect that directly affects your sex life.

A woman's body produces higher levels of oxytocin; a chemical that cancels out the effects of the sex hormone testosterone when they undergo chronic tension, as a result, their libido tends to decrease.

Even in today's progressive age, women still spend nearly an hour more each single day than men on household chores and childcare. No points for guessing, women aren't in the mood for sex because they're tired!

Chapter 2: Relating In Relationships

You're not quite sure when it happened. You used to have so much fun in bed, but now your sex life just isn't what it used to be. At night you're more interested in watching telly than indulge in a steamy session with your partner. Even when you do work up the energy, making love feels predictable.

Sex is instinctive; both men and women have certain desires and needs, sexually. It takes the absence of an interfering mind and involves overall surrender to the act and impulses of the moment.

Sow Seeds of Love

In long term relationships both partners know what turns on their partners and what puts them off. Why not reinvent what you both are comfortable with; indulge in new places, situations, lightings, simply use your imagination in alignment with your comfort level.

Make some changes to the colognes and scents you use, change the colors and textures of the tapestries in your bedroom that induce warmth and serve to rekindle your mood; get out of your regular sweat pants, and wear something revealing and sensual to feel around your skin.

Tease each other, doing this the right way can prove fruitful. Always let your partners know what feels best, if a certain move they make or a position you indulge in felt good, do communicate it to them. Expecting your partner to be a mind reader is foolish.

For many, open and direct communication in sexual matters is fraught with anxiety and fear of judgment. When urges and feelings are repressed they create emotional and sexual distance between partners.

Why wait until valentines, or birthdays and anniversaries, to express little acts of love, do small things everyday for the one you love, it could be brewing them a cup of coffee, cooking their favourite meal, or renting out your partner's favourite movie and enjoying it with them, or arranging a surprise boys night for your man, or baking a cake for your wife.

The internet is flooded with information on improving your sex life, from role playing, to bondage, to oral sex, to being sleazy and raunchy, but the fact remains that if you do not pay attention to the person you share your life with and care the least about how they feel, finding a solution through tailored sex lessons won't lead to a satisfying relationship.

A relationship is not about two bodies sweating together; it's about two people who unite as one on all levels.

Sex is a biological need, and everyone likes sex — a lot, and couples do love each other; however, there are all kinds of emotional and psychological barriers to having good sex, from poor body image to boredom.

Mind-Body-Spirit

Everything is life is interconnected. Akin to love, sex encompasses mind, body and spirit. At the very least, sex provides stress release. As you evolve psychologically, spiritually, and relation-ally you will be empowered to ascertain your true sexual self. At its peak, intimate sexual expressions can be a transcendental occurrence.

Sex becomes better as you move through life, gaining awareness, being confident and extend the capacity for emotional intimacy. Don't always wait until it's time to hit the sack. Touch each other a lot, not necessarily sexually, -- a cuddle, hugs, a pat, kisses, pecks are all ways to communicate you care.

And when a person feels desired, they feel better about themselves and this tremendously helps revive the relationship.

Self Help

Quiet your mind using therapeutic music or meditation and inquire your sexual desires. Notice negative thought patterns or beliefs and replace them with positive affirmation, understanding that primal instincts are natural. Document the issues preventing you from having a desired sex life.

Reconnect with your partner by engaging in couple activities; enjoy music together, travel, cook, and dance. Visit places you did while dating. Seek ways to deal with these issues, involve a therapist if the need arises.

Do not let days, months, and years go by before you voice out your concerns; either as an individual or as a couple. Always consult a professional if the issue has been prevailing over an extended period.

Have Mind Blowing Sex and Improve Your Relationship Forever

Don't ruin it by putting up a pirated show! Yes, we all at some point or another imitate erotic moves and positions that professional porn artists perform under the guidance of staged and scripted setups.

Let's get real, real life is not a movie, and walking around wearing 7 inch heels and being whipped is certainly not arousing, at least not for the woman. Great sex is all about comfort - physically, mentally and emotionally.

Be Imaginative

It's the weekend and you both are in front of the television after an exhausting week of work woes, it harms no one to use a little beer, or wine in moderation that helps you loosen up and cuddle together, what follows next is up to your imagination.

If you're in no mood for alcohol, share some ice-creams with chocolate sauce or a bowl of fresh juicy fruits. Don't worry about drips, pamper your partner --feeding each other can lead to a lot more. Take showers together, stock up you bathroom cabinet with aroma candles, bath oils, and lotions for a perfect sensual massage.

Are you prepared to rekindle your Passion?

Recreate your initial days together; the time you met your partner. Think about all the things you said and did for each other, no matter how silly or wildly in love things you said then.

Make up sex --after an argument, lovemaking can be extra tender and memorable.

Invest in decent nightwear, and this doesn't just apply to women, men too need to pay heed to this tip too. No one finds a person attractive walking around in ill fitted, worn out pyjamas, it's the age of the metrosexual man.

Women like well groomed men, and gone are the days when sweaty shirts and garlic breath from a man was considered normal.

Chapter 3: Tips to Make Sex Hotter and Your Relationship Happier

Here are some habits that you'd do well to adopt if you want your happily-ever-after.

- Find time to "catch up" with each other over an unhurried dinner or breakfast. Express your hopes and dreams, clear the air and you can both relax. From there, it's not such a long distance into the bedroom. Morning heavy petting can make the whole day more exciting.

- Pay attention to nerve endings, the area around the neck and shoulders, the tips of fingers, receptive spots such as the navel, the lower abdomen, the thighs and feet are very sensitive to touch and can arouse feelings of passion if caressed to pleasure. Playing some erotic music and using blindfolds will create anticipation. Tie your partner's hands and let them keep guessing about what's going to happen next. Use props to enhance the experience.

- Don't be afraid or embarrassed to try new things, if you are curious about oral sex just try it a couple of times and pay attention to how your partner feels while you're going down on them.

- Are you always up for missionary? How about you gear up on spooning or try something from the Kama-Sutra. Variety is the spice of life and variety in the bedroom can take the relationship into an entirely new dimension.

- Create an ambiance in the bedroom that inspires sensuality even after you've had a tiring day. If you're not the kinds to fuss over scented candles and soft music just use dim lights in the bedroom or around the bed. Remember less is always more. Keeping pictures of the two of you together in the bedroom is always a good reminder of the happy times you shared and helps you can go down memory lane together, reviving fond memories.

- Send each other text messages frequently. You may text your partner about general stuff on a regular day, but receiving a naughty text while you're preoccupied and in the middle of something can be a very pleasant surprise. Getting frisky over text messages proves healthy in keeping the relationship alive.

- It isn't always necessary to make love in the bedroom or the couch, or the kitchen counter, and showers. Get out of your house, take a drive to some place safe and secluded, play music, and make love. Who cares if you're married and have kids, just let go and behave like teenagers.

- Many women are out of touch with their bodies and they have no idea what to ask for. Help your partner, and yourself, by showing him what turns you on. Women who have great sex lives feel fabulous about their bodies; they see themselves as desirable and sexy. Unfortunately, research reveals 80 percent of women in the United States suffer from a negative body image. Typically, when a woman looks at herself, her eyes go straight to her problem areas and hold onto that feeling in the bedroom and when their partner's kiss their thighs or go down on them, they're busy thinking, about how ugly they look and feel embarrassed.

- To heighten your self-confidence, give yourself a reality check. The next time you're at the store or in the gym, look around you at all the women who are a variety of shapes and sizes and remind yourself: There is no one who's perfect. Talk to your partner what he loves about your body, wear clothes that enhance your assets, compliment yourself. Stand in front of the mirror naked and focus on your favourite features. Touch each part and see how you feel about it. Do something that makes you feel good in your skin at least once a day — treat yourself to a massage, use minimal make up --even if you're a stay at home mom, wear jeans or dresses that give your ego a boost, try a makeover at least once a year.

- Working out is a great way to heighten your sex life. Exercising not only strengthens the cardiovascular system, it also improves blood circulation, and gets blood flowing to all the right places. It stimulates the body, nervous system and the brain, as a result you're more physiologically excited and more receptive to sex. It also reduces stress and boosts your self-esteem and gets you in the mood. Exercising helps you tune in to your body, and force you to focus on your muscles. When your attention is entirely on yourself, you really are aware of every move, and that positions you in a better sensual state.

- Learn yoga, breathing exercises and yoga poses help release stress. Yoga helps revitalize the body and boosts stamina. Do them solo or even better if you and your partner practice it together.

- Learn to enjoy the sensuality of sex --get undressed, dim the lights, and tease yourself and your partner; take turns exploring each other's bodies. When you're the one doing the touching, deliberate on communicating love and sensuality to your partner. If you're at the receiving end, allow yourself to feel the sensations of each and every caress. This helps couples reconnect with each other on an absolutely fresh altitude. The secret is to let the anticipation build. Use your hands to guide your partner's hands in how you want to be touched — including how much pressure to exercise. When you're ready to move on to oral sex, or to use sex toys, speak up!

This is the only way your partner's going to know what turns you on.

- People can have a lot of trouble staying close; they get into relationships thinking they're automatically going to know how to make things work, but figuring out how to stay passionate together is in fact a skill --fight fair; believe it or not, learning to fight right is a key to keep chemistry alive. There doesn't exist, a relationship without disagreements, but when there is an understanding that your partner can come to you with any disagreement without being attacked, you will have an honest relationship embracing open discussions in replacement of fights.

- Most importantly remember your wedding vows. You may have trouble over years with the person you promised to love and to honour and cherish till death do you part, life happened and things came in the way. Sex is an expression of love, ignite love by all means, and stop worrying about how to be good at sex. Mind-blowing sex follows when you look beyond each other's flaws and stop comparing your life with the lives of those who you think are ideal.

Chapter 4: Healthy Lifestyle and Sex

Welcome to the fourth chapter of this book. Here we are going to walk you through the various lifestyle choices that an average person ignores and blatantly un-follows thereby bringing upon himself a series of health adversities, and eventually, sex issues.

This chapter contains a summary of all the changes you could start making to your life that will lead you to experience a healthy sex life for a period longer than you would have otherwise. We are all blessed with a specific amount of lifetime on this planet. Some people survive longer than the rest, while some give up the battle midway.

On top of this unequal distribution of lifetime, we end up inviting external causes of life-degradation, forcing our already negligible life span to get further reduced by significant margins. Enlisted below are some of the significant changes that you need to usher into your life so as to expect your sex lives to spice up along with it:

Eat Healthy

Do not neglect what goes into your body. In order for your sexual glands to function at their optimum levels, it is highly vital that your body receives the required amount of proteins, carbohydrates, fats and minerals and vitamins.

Try to replace your old diet with a balanced diet that contains all the necessary ingredients in the appropriate proportions. Instead of opting for junk food for evening snacks, prefer something homemade. Do not eat an excess of a single ingredient and try to even it out with the other ingredients in case you have consumed one ingredient in abundance.

One very vital factor in sexual performance is the rate of blood flow in your body. The higher the rate the better your performance. In human males, the pace in which blood is pumped to the genitals is detrimental in how good their sex lives are.

The blood vessels around your genitals perform a crucial function in giving you the ultimate pleasure during a sexual act. When you are 'in the mood', your blood vessels fire up and the blood flow to your sexual glands is at its peak. It is primarily due to the blood rushing into them that you get 'excited' and 'ready' for some 'action'.

It has been scientifically proven that vegetables like onion, beetroots and radishes improve your blood flow and increase your hemoglobin count. Consumption of such vegetables will eventually lead you to have a sex life that has been naturally enhanced and not artificially helped.

Stay Fit

A lot of people confuse fitness with bodybuilding. This myth needs to be done away with. The difference between staying fit and staying ripped is a major one.

For a healthy sex life, you need to stay fit, nothing else. Fitness is acquired when your body is at peace with you. It is that state of your physical state when all your body parts are not just functioning well, but also giving you satisfaction by their work.

For example, if you have a weak spine you will face problems bending down to pick up a pen. However, if it is in great shape, probably due to you hitting the gym, you won't face any issue doing simple things like bending down for a pen.

Being physically fit is a major advantage for people looking forward to spice up their sex lives. What more could a partner want than a body that is in perfect shape, built by months or years of going to the gym and jogging the field. A fit body is a desirable body.

Even during the real 'act', a fit body is able to sustain more than an unfit one. It all comes down to performance for the main act. If you are physically weak, you will end up disappointing your partner when it comes to performing some daring moves.

Here are some life-changing tips to stay fit throughout the year:

- Eat a balanced diet; one which comprises of all ingredients in proportional amounts.

- Get up early in the morning to jog around the local park.

- Hit the gym and start working out so as to keep your body in shape.

- Quit food that is rich in fat, carbs and too much

unsaturated fat. Not only do you have to eat healthy, but you will also have to cut down on food that is harmful to your body. Try to also quit junk food, if you are into the habit of consuming them even for light snacks.

- Do not overstretch yourself trying to become an alpha male. Yes, physical fitness is desirable. Yes, a good body is what gets you all the attention. But a good physique is not the be-all and end-all of a good sex life. Surely, having a good body is an edge but if you over do it, or push for it too much, you won't be doing yourself a favor.

- For the purpose of the above-mentioned point, make an agenda of working out so you don't end up trying to overreach. Sit down with your private trainer at the gym, and chalk out your weekly schedule of working out. Make a list of all the exercises that you would be able to do and all those you wouldn't be. Do not hesitate to tell your trainer about your bodily limitations and weaknesses. It is important that you become honest with the one person who is in charge of transforming your physique. By doing so you ensure that the final plan that gets chalked out for you is something suitable for you and not according to an ideal body person.

Positive Attitude

Yes, you read that right. How you think does affect how you perform in bed. A positive attitude refers to that state of mind, which is inducing of happy thoughts, positive ideas and creative inputs- all signs of a flourishing and running mental state.

Let us figure out how a good state of mind could be possibly related to your sex life.

James is an investment banker at a prestigious bank in the city. His wife, Katherine, is a household manager. James' sex life has been right on track until he started getting flak for his shortcomings in the office. He started sulking because of the failures he faced at work and no longer had breakfast at home before heading out for the office.

He replaced his cell phone number with a new one and started going out with colleagues lesser than what he used to. He would now ignore his wife and instead the only free time he got was at the house, to do office work, trying to meet new deadlines.

The issues that James faced at work have now started affecting his personal, and to be more specific, his sexual life. Katherine and James do not indulge themselves in carnal pleasures anymore. Katherine, who used to be a regular follower of monthly precautions taken in the form of habitual pills, is now off of them. It is so because there is no longer any sort of intimacy between her and her husband.

The above illustration just goes to show that a positive attitude is supremely vital to a good sex life. It may not directly affect how you perform in bed, but it will have an important say in deciding your build-up mood that comes before even the thought of sex creeps into your mind.

When you are stressed, your mind shuts itself off to any suggestions of recreation. Sex is one of them. You are just too engrossed in trying to figure out ways out of your life's problems to be able to divert your mind to something so basic and so humane in nature- sex.

You slowly start ignoring an important aspect of your life. You no longer play the role of the loving husband and have turned into a machine that travels to work, comes home to sleep and eats somewhere in the middle.

Happiness

Happiness is both- the cause and result of sex. It is very natural to understand as to why it's a result. However, the role of happiness as a cause for sex can be understood in layers. First you have to grasp the concept that when the human mind is in a state of bliss, it tends to be more productive and more fun loving.

There are no inhibitions put on it regarding what it can and cannot do. The happier you stay in your life, the better your sex life is going to get. It is a simple equation.

Freedom from Stress

Stress is that looming cloud over everything good happening in your life, that rains heavily without warning. The world is a huge rat race and we are all rats competing in it, running without clue, searching for the elusive trophy.

The cycle of survival has pushed us humans to forget the bare essentials of living and compelled us to seek something that is superficial, temporary and tempting. We no longer find pleasure in reading a book, watching a movie or hanging out with buddies. Simple activities have been replaced by commercialized ones.

We are more concerned about the economy than the community. We would rather go visit a mall than enjoy a stroll in the park. Life has become so success-and-material oriented that we are getting more and more detached from genuine happiness.

We struggle to meet deadlines and get pushed into stress when we fail. Stress therefore, is always on the prowl, waiting on the edge, for you to fail. Stress has become common and it's gained an inevitable role in our lives. Be it the office work or the household chores, we manage to track down stress and beg it to occupy its supreme position in our schedule.

It has now been ingrained into human nature to obsess over things that rarely matter. We stress out over things that are not worth it.

The more engrossed you will remain in stress, the more degrading your sex life will become. Sex is about liberating yourself and letting go of all inhibitions. It is about connecting with an individual on such a supreme level that you entirely forget anything else for those sweaty thirty minutes (or less or more!).

Stress doesn't kill your mood; it never lets it take birth. Freedom from stress is another way to improve your sex life. Try to take matters that are not worth your attention, in a lighter vein. Do not over-think about people, their judgments and the consequences of ignoring them. Have confidence in your individualism and its power to drive away the negativity others throw at you.

Chapter 5: Variety is the Spice of Life

The human mind is fantastically imaginative. When you think about how to cook noodles, it will come up with approximately eight different ways and seventeen different ingredients to spice it up for a memorable experience. When you think about what to wear on a fancy occasion, it will conjure up so many different ideas on what cloth to opt for, what fabric to choose, which accessories will make your outfit extraordinary and what colors will make your eyes pop.

In so many such endeavors in everyday life, your brain starts whirling into action, and your heart starts pumping faster. The fact of the matter is that we, as humans, strive to bring variety into our lives.

Our entire body follows our wonderfully imaginative brain into the playground and complies happily to all the fantasies being cooked up in our minds. The telltale signs being heavier breathing and faster heartbeat. Our innermost thoughts themselves seem to glow with the prospect of something more exciting and more fulfilling.

Why wouldn't we, then, obvious that one of the most intimate activities that our bodies are hardwired to do, will entail such thorough weaving of imagination from our minds?

Sex is the most primal activity in our lives. It's utterly natural that we would want to make it more exciting and filled with wonderment. Yes, you might enjoy the good ol' vanilla sex, but it is called 'vanilla' for a reason.

Generally vanilla is an aphrodisiac flavor and appealing to our tastes, but at the end of the day it can turn into one of the most bland and boring flavors to our taste buds. Imagine going to a restaurant and ordering the same dish over and over again. Yes, the cook might change every few months but the spices wouldn't. Supply of the same spices every time you crave some food, will leave your palate awfully unsatisfied and bored!

The restaurant metaphor heavily resounds with your sex life. Missionary may feel great for some time, but the eventual rhythmic thrusting day in and day out will leave either or both of you severely bored. And well, sex should be anything but boring.

It should leave you breathless and craving for more. It is then essential to unleash the inner devils and goddesses in you; thereby filling your sex lives with renewed amazement.

You might have been craving to try that mischievous doggy position you have always wondered about, or you might have researched a new mysterious position that hasn't left your imagination for five weeks now. Whatever the scenario might be, it will help you if you shed your awkward inhibitions and went ahead and talked to your partner about it.

With an understanding partner, the most probable outcome would be that they would want to try out the same thing with you. Plus, the added bonus of guiding them through the process will put you into the front seat and add that extra oomph in your sex drive. You won't even realize but the vanilla would have changed into a chocolate, with a tang of strawberry and a boost of vodka!

If you've already tried all the feasible positions in the great book of sex and are still craving for more variety, don't worry; there is a plethora of activities that can be incorporated in your sex lives. Each serving on the platter more arousing and erotic than the next.

Some people don't like being in the front seat. They prefer being on their knees instead. Probably one of the most widely famous sex patterns all around the world, this puts one of the partners in the dominant position and the other partner in the meek position of a submissive.

The details and the extent of contribution to the activity is mutually decided. The submissive will feel pleasantly naughty catering to the whim and fancy of the dominant; while giving up control, both physical and mental.

The dominant will experience sweet satisfaction in exploring and playing with their partners. Both the participants thoroughly enjoy the role-play and it can be immensely satisfying.

Many other forms of role-play can be key erotic elements in your sex life. The combination of fantasy mixed with reality can be an intoxicating drug. Always imagined being a rescuer to a stranded damsel in distress? Or wanted to be frisked by a macho looking civil officer?

Incorporating elaborate role-play into your bedroom might

soothe those fluttering butterflies in your stomach. Seeing your loving partner in such tempting backdrops will send your loins into a frenzy and the sex will be even more pleasurable. It will pacify all those fantasies you might have had while watching a surreal movie or while surfing the internet.

Not only these, there is an abundance of ventures that can be explored. Having been recently discovered and utilized, the use of suitable objects according to individual needs and imaginations has become a popular affair with many.

Aptly named as 'sex toys', these devices are primarily used to facilitate human sexual pleasure. People engaging in regular sex might find these little ornaments to be most gratifying. These are available in such a huge range that often, a person finds themselves spoilt for choice.

We recommend you to try as many of these playthings as your heart desires. Vibrator wands are often welcome with women. Whether in the company of a partner or while enjoying some alone time, the use of these wonderfully magical dildos can push a woman's pleasure to heightened peaks and deliver them to a blissful state through the big 'O' gate.

More famous sex toys can include penile rings, or harnesses for men. These can help simulate both the partners during sexual intercourse. Other raunchy penetrative toys may include anal beads or butt plugs for the extra boost to the traditional 'vanilla' sex.

One or both partners often enjoy the erotic component introduced by the implementation of these sex toys. And the physical ecstasy often renders them content and pleased.

You can also opt to go for a different route, and we mean literally. Greed is the one thing primal with all humans. And why not? There's no harm in yearning for more indulgence. Often frolicking around in the conventional playground leaves the participants craving for more.

These needs can be easily met when there is another tunnel around the playground, which can make the ride seem even more enjoyable!

A score of kink enthusiasts often luxuriate themselves with anal sex, which is the act in which an erect penis is inserted into a person's anus for sexual pleasure. With mutual understanding and love, this activity brings continual delectation to the 'performing' partner and the recipient of the passionate thrusts often reports a pleasurable feeling of fullness and satisfaction.

Engaging yourself in a loving manner with your partner will bring the joy and charm into your relationship that you've always wanted and wondered about.

That being said, there is no rigid set of points to be followed. The boundaries of exploring your partners are ever expanding. The basic aim is to please yourself and your partner without bending to any particular social stigma. What happens in the privacy of a bedroom will define your mental and emotional state in life.

Your instincts should drive you. Your spirit shouldn't subdue any wild torrent of kinks. Instead, shedding the awkward inhibitions and embracing the beauty of the human body will bring you to a delicious state of nirvana.

Chapter 6: Foreplay

Human bodies are one of the most complex things ever created on this planet. There are plenty of processes that turn this elemental structure into a sophisticated and pristine machine. Many life processes, muscles, tissues and organs work in harmony to make us who we are. Every organ has its own need and every process requires thorough preparation.

Digestion needs proper food. Respiration needs breathable air. Similarly, circulation needs viable energy. All these life processes need resources of their own. Reproduction requires a different kind of need and preparation.

As humans, our minds are hardwired to think and imagine. And our bodies are made to feel and experience. Combine these elements into one package, and viola! You have the key to a spiritual and happy life, and sex is one of the most primal needs of life.

Pleasurable sex is what all humans in this world aim for. The ultimate satisfaction from delightful sex is hardly ever beaten by anything else. Then, it should come as no surprise, that people go to all kinds of lengths to fulfill their partners sexually, thereby fulfilling other physical and emotional needs.

The average crowd that actively participates in sexual activities often tends to jump the queue and skip to the generic thrusting and pumping. Although it might feel satisfying on some level, it will never feel blissfully gratifying as when you incorporate some basic tricks from this book.

The attention to detail and technicality, in itself, can greatly enhance boring intercourse. By brushing this off as a mere a triviality, you might be eluding yourself and your partner from that heart-thumping, mind-blowing release.

Extending the Foreplay

Deriving from the name itself, 'fore' meaning 'before something', foreplay is like a prelude to a play, a trailer to a movie or more aptly, an appetizer to a main course. Without a prelude, even a wonderful play will seem uninteresting; a great movie will have no audience and a main course will seem unfinished and unappetizing.

When everyday trivial tasks will seem bland and mundane without a proper foreword, then it doesn't require one to be a rocket-scientist to figure out that a highly important task of intercourse will need a tantalizingly tempting foreplay.

Just like a hot soup will increase your craving for the subsequent lamb, a slow tease into the main intercourse will multiply your appetite for it.

There are many ways of enhancing the experience of sexual intercourse. Men and women both, can include these tricks into their sexual lives. Even though men and women think differently, the basic need is to heighten the lust in the relationship, leading to a great and extended sexual release.

Pleasing a Man

Men are very visual when it comes to their sex lives. Their minds take a backseat and their vision predominates the way to their heart. In order to satisfy a man in foreplay, very basic details need to be followed.

Men love it when a lot is left to their imagination. They love to be teased and tantalized with. They will rarely admit to it, but they love the initial chase. And nothing screams 'chase' more than a sexy striptease. You can wear the most ravishing outfit you own and strut in front of your partner to stir their imagination.

Their hearts will already be fluttering by now. Careful as to not rush it, sway to the rhythm of the music or their strum of fingers in anticipation. Make it as visually appealing as possible.

Shed the outfit in unnervingly slow movements, alluring them into the tease. Carried out with teasing vivaciousness, it will leave your man filled with jaw dropping anticipation and thinking 'what's next?'

There is a very systematic way with which men can be aroused. A gentle brush of hands here and a lingering touch there, will leave them wanting for much more. The art of using your hand can be of great help here. The accurate nooks and crevices stroked with the precise pressure can be heavily stimulating.

Not only the right amount of pressure, but it is essential to maintain a continual rhythm and to not let it dissipate. Rhythmic strokes can help build the excitement and further the jubilation.

The most important and significant part in foreplay for men goes to the tactful and skillful usage of tongue and mouth. We have already established that men are very visual in nature. And at the end of the day they are nothing but slaves to their carnal desires if the right buttons are pushed.

They are sinfully naughty in their minds and would love for those thoughts to transform into reality. All men love their manhood, they have been self-taught into loving it since puberty. And they know it feels good to bring their lust into fruition. So, when they see their partners show that much adoration and care for their loins, their lust exalts. This is the base of foreplay for them.

Most positions work for a proper 'blowjob'. All men are different in that way. Some like to be in a more physically relaxed lying down state, while others might like to stand and enjoy the view from above. It will all boil down to how seductively and alluringly you can draw out the process, scientifically called fellatio.

Male genitalia is filled with nerve endings, which will experience a rush of blood circulation when touched temptingly. And that is what the aim is. You can incorporate as many newer and fancier techniques you want, but the basic pressure and moisture that your mouth will serve, will have no match to almost anything.

Many men report to feel pure bliss when they feel the warmth and coziness of a tongue sliding over their member. Their loins are sure to go into a tizzy and leave them with pure carnal joy.

More can be explored with men, each preference varying with each couple; the elemental desire remains the same. Physical satisfaction will make them joyous and they are sure to deliver the pleasure back with an excitement and rejuvenated vigor.

Pleasing a Woman

Women are slightly different from men when it comes to foreplay. Women are not as visual as men are. The wires from their eyes to their groin are not as securely connected as they are in men. Rarely can a woman be aroused by a tantalizing lap dance.

Yes, they may enjoy the show and appreciate the effort being put into it, but they will not quite experience the stir 'down there' as a man might do when used like a chair or a pole for a lap-dance.

A woman is like soup on a cold wintry day. Soup has the potential of warming you up and providing you with a passionate glow on a cold bleak day. It can work wonders to your body and leave you completely fulfilled. But like a bored woman, cold soup will leave you shivery and anguished and will not help in perking your day up.

Soup needs to be warmed up from within so that it can be properly relished. And similarly, a woman needs to be shown care and adoration for her to properly fulfill your desires.

The thing to be remembered is that each woman is different in her own way. There is no systematic set of instructions that can be followed here, as in the case of men. Different women crave touches in different places with varying pressure and rhythm. But when shown meticulous care and attention, they can be satiated and left craving for more.

The basic mental stimulant of a woman lies in her mind. If you can grasp the attention of her mind, you are all the more closer to satisfy her need. Melodious music can tingle at her psyche and heighten her curiosity and sense of excitement.

Most women value cleanliness and will definitely appreciate romantic surroundings. Scented candles and ambient lighting might grasp her attention much more than a spotless and textured tie around your neck. Paying attention to these seemingly trivial details will help you a long way to a home run.

You may start with lighter and softer touches. Lingering them feather-like all over her body and finding those sweet spots where she will evidently enjoy sensations, are the first few steps in firing her up.

Showering attention on her breasts is another sure-shot step towards the goal. The mammary glands in women are filled with nerve endings and teasing these will leave a sauntering effect on her body.

Many a time, body parts like thighs and the neck are ignored in the rush to hit 'Australia' down there. This could easily be a gross misstep. The region around the neck for women is very sensitive and any slight touch can make it tingly and arousing. Similarly, body areas like inner thighs and back, when caressed with precision can bring immense joy.

Some women may prefer their toes being cuddled and some may like their naval being fondled. A sensual touch on an accurate point is sure to have her moan out loud. You only need to figure out which embrace triggers her excitement and which fizzles out.

Finally, after potentially warming her up, you can aim to push her to the precipice. You may use your expert fingers into skillfully exploring the cave. If you have done all the steps before this correctly, you will find that your touch encounters almost no friction during the exploration. You may further enhance the smoothness of the cruise by stroking her in all the correct directions.

The use of your tongue will come in great assistance to your advantage here. The tongue as a muscle can bend in ways no other body part in a human can bend. And this little fact can come in handy while remembering to pleasure your partners.

Not only will it feel overtly pleasurable but also very special. Just the feeling of being appreciated in that intimate way is sure to make the woman in your life positively beaming with delight.

The Key Lies In....

The key to a great foreplay lies in the premise that both the partners should thoroughly enjoy being with each other. Half of the pleasure is often derived from the knowledge that your partner is being pleased with the efforts you have put in.

You might have researched articles or thoroughly read this book to seamlessly incorporate these methods into your sex life. After going to such great lengths with the sole intention of fulfilling your partner's desire at heart, seeing the efforts come into fruition will bring utter jubilance to you.

So, if you like a certain technique or an enrapturing touch, your partner would love to hear your moans and grunts arising from pure carnal pleasure. Foreplay is an intimate activity that brings the partners closer to each other, both physically and mentally.

It should be embraced with the reverence and adoration of mature and understanding individuals. And then you'll be just mere bystanders as you witness the excitement and rigor in your sex life shoot up and out to the heavens.

Chapter 7:
Sexual Positions

Welcome to the seventh chapter of this book. Here comes the interesting part of this whole journey. You will be made familiar with various innovative and different positions that you may try out with your partners in order to spice up your sex life.

As mentioned in the fifth chapter, everyone loves a little variety in their life. No one likes to get stuck with 'vanilla' their whole life. Everyone wants to explore more flavors, find new avenues, hunt for more exciting prospects. This leads to couples trying out new methods of lovemaking.

The missionary position's value starts degrading after the first few times, your genitals scream for more exciting positions to be tried.

Enlisted below are some of the unconventional positions we would advise you to try in case your sex life has spiraled down towards monotonousness.

Anal

Clearly, the most unconventional of the positions, the Anal or the Doggy position requires the woman partner to get on all fours and try to push out her hips as much as she can. The pushing of the hips is necessary so as to make it easier for the man to enter her with comfort.

The man goes behind the woman, gets on his own knees, and places his erect member on the entrance of the 'back door'. After caressing the backdoor with his fingers for a while (so that the 'door' is well prepared), he can start taking mild thrusts into her with his penis.

It is not easy for couples who have never done it, to try it for the first time. It can get quite painful for the female partner hence it is advised for the male to take care that there is enough lubrication used, natural or otherwise.

Cowgirl

You must be familiar with the term if you are a regular subscriber of unconventional sites. The male partner lies down on the floor with his member in a fully attentive position. The female partner's function lies in spreading her legs while standing right above the male partner who is lying down on the floor.

With spread legs, she is to slowly 'sit' on the member, while trying to ease the member into her. After the easing has been accomplished, the female partner is to fold her knees and assume a sitting position on her male partner who is still lying down.

With power accumulated from the folded knees, which are now used as support, she is to perform a squatting exercise of sorts so as to thrust herself into the penis by bouncing up and down.

Reverse Cowgirl

The reverse cowgirl is the exact opposite of cowgirl. Literally so. While in cowgirl, the female partner faces the male partner, i.e., their faces are opposite of each other.

In reverse cowgirl position, the girl faces the male partner's legs and lets him enjoy the sweet scenery of her backside. The reverse cowgirl position is a clear favourite of many males because of the following reasons:

One, it lets them have a good spectacle of their female partners' butts. Nothing turns on a man like a shapely butt during thrusting. Trust me on this, a nice butt when seen from the angle the male partner in the reverse cowgirl sees, is a gift from the gods.

Second, it lets the male partner relax a bit. It is natural that they would enjoy a position that requires minimal effort from their end.

Scissors

As the name suggests, both partners have to be physically so aligned as to give the impression of a pair of scissors at work. The female partner lies down with her legs spread, the right leg spread in the upward direction with the left lying still.

By now, the male partner is prepared to diagonally enter the female partner with his penis thrusting forward. The only difference between this position and the missionary position is that missionary is straight out entering while this replies more on the position of legs. The legs are so aligned that both the pairs seem to have crossed each other, as if trying to cut.

The Sultry Saddle

For this one, you will have to work out your imagination. The phrase 'Sultry Saddle' should give you some idea about the operation of this position.

The male partner lies down with his penis at full attention. The female eases herself on the attentive penis while sliding down her left leg under his and keeping her right leg intact. There is a crisscross situation so formed now.

The female starts rocking herself on the partner while grabbing the male partner by his chest. This whole picture is that of a female riding a horse, which explains the name.

The Cradle

In this case, the name won't be helpful for you to guess the working of the position. Let me explain how this operates. The male partner sits in a cross-legged position with his penis ready.

The female partner does the same, except additionally she also moves on top of the male partner, without the male partner having to lie down. Now both the partners are sitting in a 'locked' position. The female is on top of the male sans the male having to get on his back. After having assumed this position, the male starts rocking forward and backward, thereby giving the impression of a cradle.

The Standing Sally

Another very erotic position many couples find exciting is the standing position. The female partner stands with her bum out while her hands rest on the wall. Her face remains firm fixated on the wall, with her butt protruding outside for the male to get aroused by.

The male stands just behind the female partner while trying to find the right 'door'. From here, the male has two choices- the front or the back door. Some males enjoy the front door while others the backdoor. It is up to the woman to decide.

The Spider

Imagine the two partners lying on their backs, with their bodies horizontally opposite of each other. Now imagine them spreading their legs and bringing them to a position from where they are able to crisscross the legs so as to give the impression of a four legged spider.

The genitals can indulge in their play from hereon while the legs relax and contract according to the intensity, frequency and passion of the thrusts.

I hope you enjoyed and learned from this chapter. We all require changes in our lives to keep us refreshed and going. Sex life can get dull after a while if you don't work at it. There are many ways to bring back the charm, and one of them is experimentation.

When you experiment with your bodies, as you used to while you were in the teenage phase, you end up realizing that there was so much more you had not explored. You will reach the epiphany that your body is a hidden chest of treasure and you have discovered only half of it.

So, indulge in new techniques of happiness and surprise yourself and more importantly, your partner. Your sex life need not be all 'vanilla'; pour in a few drops of chocolate too and witness the taste getting better every day.

Chapter 8:
Revival of the Sex Drive

Welcome to the chapter whose title is one of the most underestimated topics when people talk about sex. Here, we shall discuss those irrelevant seeming things that are of supreme importance but are often swept under the rug, overshadowed by more important aspects of the game.

Sex is divine. Yes, nothing connects two people like sex does. When your partner understands, caring and willing for experimentation, your sex life is bound to improve and stay fresh all the time.

But what if things aren't all roses all the time? What if you are stuck with a partner who has grown out of the honeymoon phase? What if you, the reader, is a middle age man who has lost all interest in bedroom activities and no longer enjoys sex as an activity? Let us try to find some answers.

Imagine coming home from work everyday, dropping your shoes at the doorstep, having a cold dinner and going to bed early. An ideal corporate life consists of exactly the same routine. Most of us mortals are trapped in the aforementioned rat race of life. We scarcely get the time to even notice our partner who's been craving for our attention all this while.

Notice

The first and foremost thing you need to do so as to start improving your sex life is to start noticing your partner. It could be anything from their new make up to a fresh pair of jeans they might have bought in order to impress you.

When you notice your partner, and their efforts to make themselves look good for you, it assures them that you guys still have the magic going on. If you ignore your partner's attempts at enhancing your sex life, they are going to completely shut themselves down after trying for a while.

It will be too late by the time you realize you need to pay them some attention. Hence, the first step to revive your dull sex life is to start paying your partner the much-deserved attention!

Compliment

Do not be shy in complimenting your partner. She bought a new pair of lingerie to please you at night, but you refuse to notice it, let alone praise it; that's what kills the charm. Noticing is not sufficient. You need to follow it up with your words.

Compliment your partner's efforts or at least acknowledge them. Do not be hesitant about saying a few words of gratitude to your partner if they have gone the extra mile to please you in the bedroom. When you express the feeling that you are awed by their experiment, they will get the confidence to try more and try better. Do not be a negative force in the relationship and gun down a bad experiment.

Care

Many partners assume care to be synonymous with care and affection. The myth needs to be stopped from getting propagated. Your care for your partner need not be out of love or romantic feelings towards them. Caring for someone should be genuine and as straight as an arrow.

Obviously, having been together for so long, you must have

developed an inherent sense of unparalleled care for your partner, the kind you would not be able to develop even for your kids. Try to revive this care.

It is when partners stop caring that issues crop up in relationships. Caring for your partner is proof that you are still present in the relationship and are willing to be more so.

Gestures

You cannot barge into the house after work, pick up your partner and start banging them and call it your sex life. No, sex life is more about loving your partner than doing your partner. Love dries up after a while. But if you try hard enough, it won't.

You could continue doing all those little things for your partner that brought you two together in the first place. Every relationship is based on some little things that both the partners have witnessed or gone through together. When you have found your bundle of little things, try to hold on to them for as long as possible.

For example, the first time you met your partner, they

were trying hard to get into a movie hall ticket's line and you helped her by offering her your place in the long line.

You could reanimate the scene by taking her to the same move hall and redoing the whole thing once again. It would be childish and sweet. Small gestures like this go a long way in cementing the relationship and prevent it from breaking apart.

The very point of this chapter is that sex is more than what happens in the bedroom. It could be happening right now, as you would be thinking of your partner while reading this chapter. It happens in the kitchen when you hold her from behind and peck on her cheeks to thank her for the awesome barbecue that she fed you for the Sunday lunch.

It could happen in a family gathering while you two are trying to find some alone time but are unable to do so because of the presence of a lot of relatives. The excitement, build up and passion parts of sex are as important as the main act itself.

You need not have sex twice a day to keep your sex life up and running. Even once a week is enough if you are doing it right and neither of the partner's is unhappy with it.

What happens in the bedroom consists of only half the experience we call sex. What happens elsewhere is the other half. You need to be in constant connection of your partner in order to fully satisfy them sexually.

Do not forget to keep teasing them whatever work you are busy with. Remember to call them at least once a day, however busy you are. Such simple things have a nice impact on your sex life. You won't notice it over night but in the long run, it will have its say.

Chapter 9:
Points to be Notes

Welcome to the ninth and the penultimate chapter of this book. As opposed to the previous chapters where you were briefed about the various ways in which you could spice up your sex life, this chapter focuses more on the attitude-aspect of sex.

It will talk about the various changes you need to bring in your behavioral and mental realms while indulging in or discussing sex with your partner.

Point of Focus

It is the unspoken duty of a partner to make it all about the other partner. Do not try to focus all your energy upon your own body. Try to regulate your energy and activity in such a manner that your partner feels craved and lusty. If all you think about and pay attention to is your own self, your partner might lose any further interest in the act. Make it a point to make the whole deal the-other-partner-oriented.

Passion

Do not climb into the bed like a zombie and start humping like corpses who have been reanimated using voodoo. Know that it's another person and they have their own tastes, likes, arousal points and sensitiveness. Realize that they need to be 'worked' before you could gain the right to go hump them like a savage.

Mix a little bit, no, a lot of passion in your bed activities. Show your partner that you are as horny as they are. Even if you are tired from work, do not hold back from releasing the beast within when it comes to performing in bed.

Performance Pressure

It is completely natural for sexual partners to feel the pressure of performance, especially during the few initial times. Sexual performance pressure is the anxiety and burden a sexual partner feels in terms of their capability, endurance and longevity in the bedroom. It is a more common phenomenon in males than it is in females.

When people feel the pressure of performance in bed, it pushes them further down. It is like quick sand; the more you dabble in it the more it pulls you down.

Here is something you need to keep in mind in case you are anticipating performance pressure related anxiety attacks- it does not matter in the end. All that does matter is how much pleasure both of you derive out of it, which becomes kind of difficult when all you have going on in your head is the surmounting pressure of it all. Do not crumble under the pressure; instead, rise stronger and harder than before.

Discomfort

Sexual discomfort could come in various forms. Sexual discomfort could arise out of a partner not feeling like having sex tonight, or one of the partners being sexually drained for a session. It could also arise from a partner being abused or made to forcefully do something in sex, that they have no taste for.

Some partners are not very comfortable with trying out 'new' positions. For example, a partner's anus may be unsuitable for anal indulgence and their previous experiences with the position may have gone bad. When forced into repeating it, they might turn hostile and get uncomfortable in the middle of the act.

Another thing that women do not particularly like is oral sex. Oral sex can be described as the taking into your mouth of sexual glands of your partner. Due to obvious reasons, many partners are not very fond of it. If such a partner is forcibly made to perform or indulge oneself in oral sex, the experience can be scary for them.

Prior bad sexual experiences also leave some people vulnerable to further wounds that are mental in nature. Make sure that besides being a great partner in bed, you are also considerate of your partner's feelings and state of mind. Do not simply impose sex on your partner. Ensure their consent and enjoyment.

In case you see any signs of discomfort displaying themselves, stop any sexual activity you are into and withdraw yourself from arousal. I know it sounds very weirdly difficult to simply 'withdraw oneself from arousal' but with sufficient willpower it can be done.

Sensual not sexy

Many couples forget the importance of sensual and try to

look for the sexy. There is a very big difference between sensual and sexy. Sexy encompasses notions of sleaziness and abundance. On the other hand, sensual is not direct and often leaves a lot to imagination.

Sensual is often preferred over sexy when it comes to going for a class act. Make sure whatever sexual activities happen between you and your partner; it falls under the category of sensual and not sexy. Sexy is good too, but sensual has got more passion and intensity to it. The level of enjoyment one might get from sensual is incomparable to the level one achieves through sexy.

The After-Sex Talk

What you do during sex is as important as what you do after it. You are a couple. That means it's two individuals that have come together to form a bond. It is a coming together of two opinions and difference of experiences are bound to arise.

A couple that stays up and talks after sex is a couple upon which an average marriage counselor would put his money on. When you talk after sex, it shows that you care for your partner. It displays your attitude that, to you, your partner is more than just a person to have frick-frack with.

It also denotes that you care enough for the partner to ask them about their experience. This behavior is not only a good tool for enhancement in relationship but also considered a hallmark of gentle-manliness.

The whole point of this chapter is that sex extends its boundaries to beyond the bed. It is not enough that you stick it in, rock back and forth, spill yourself inside and get done with it. Various humane elements also form parts of the human sex life. One must focus more on improving one's sex life rather than sex drive. Sex drive can be worked upon, medically or otherwise. But a great sex life is often hard to achieve, and in extreme cases, regain.

Once gone, a good sex life proves hard to return. One must always strive to keep oneself sexually active. There should be no set time for engaging oneself in naughty works of the bedroom. Do not make sex a routine affair. You would be making a major blunder by setting a schedule for having sex.

The very nature of sex dictates that it should be

spontaneous and random. Your life would be boring, dull, and repetitive if you perform sex as just another duty. Indulge in the act as if your life depends on it. Do it as if the world is going to end tomorrow and the next are the only moments left to live.

Make sure your partner and you enjoy the best of each other. Do not give your partner any reason to get put off by anything you do during the act.

Know your partner inside out. By doing so you have gained enough knowledge about their likes, dislikes, tastes and distastes. It so follows that you are no longer a stranger to your partner and are hence at a better position to know what's going on. This way, whenever they have a problem related to your sexual life, you will be the first to know.

Lack of communication even in the matter of sex can result disastrously for you. Make sure even during the performance of the 'act', you two keep talking. Reach an agreement regarding 'stop words'.

Some couples use 'stop words' to communicate. The idea behind having a stop word is to let the partner know when the act is becoming painful or uncomfortable.

It may so happen that a couple is role-playing and the word 'stop' or 'no' gets used as part of the role-playing. Such a scenario partners wouldn't know when the other partner is being themselves and when they are playing the part. For such circumstances, agree on a random word to be allowed the status of the stop word, which when used would signal red.

The entire point of sex is to attain pleasure. If by any way, be it intentional or otherwise, one or both the partners are unable to do that, it means the process needs to be restarted again, the clocks need to be rewound and the wheels need to be brought back to their original position.

Sex is a beautiful activity. It is meant to be enjoyed and experimented with. It is like an unknown wood, which you stumble upon while out on a picnic. The more you walk into it, the more it fascinates you.

Chapter 10:
Eroticism

There are many instances throughout a day when only a couple of your senses are heightened. Human beings are typically said to have five senses. The sense of vision, the sense of smell, the sense of taste, the sense of hearing and the sense of touch.

An average human will mostly neglect one or two of these senses in their everyday tasks. How grossly unfair is it! Imagine going to an unlimited buffet and having to pay for a full plate but only relishing one or two of the dishes. It can seem not only disappointing but also unsatisfying.

Or imagine going fishing, catching a fish that is only large in size but not appealing to the sense of smell or touch. How unappetizing it can be! Similarly, imagine attending a widely popular musical show on Broadway. But what if your eyes were blindfolded or your ears were plugged shut? Wouldn't being restricted of that one very essential sense leave you frustrated and annoyed?

Unappetizing sex is not unlike all these frustrating

experiences. Following some techniques and definitive movements with proper friction and velocity forms the essence of the actual deed of sexual intercourse.

But there can be a lot more perspectives to the act of lovemaking. Those that should not be neglected no matter how petty they may sound.

Eroticism is the generic quality of being capable of having sexual feelings by not just the basic art of sex, by tugging at the many psychological and philosophical aspects of the human mind. This tends to draw the focus on the aesthetics of sexual desire, the sensuality of seduction, and the romance of ravishing intercourse.

Different people have their brains wired differently. And eroticism is mostly dependent on a person's individual morality. Some people get attracted by the intoxicating aroma of freshly shampooed hair or the pleasant fragrances wafting from their partners after a refreshing bath or the cozy warmth emanating after the bathroom has been freshly used for a hot shower.

Other people may get turned on by an elaborate display of erotic artwork or the harmonic resonance of a powerful piece of music. You can also find posing in front of your partner lying down on a couch while they may photograph you with raw sensual desire highly appealing.

This may seem like a clichéd scene from a popular movie, but clichés work, and that is why they are named so.

In this age and time, when working for a regular income is one of the most essential ways of leading a comfortable life, hectic days accompany desirable salaries like creaking doors accompany haunted houses. Then, who wouldn't welcome a sensual back rub or head massage from their loving partners after such a hectic day.

After spending an entire day pushing against deadlines, an erotic oil massage over their limbs and loins will bring soothing peace and gratification to your partners. This is basically what erotica aims at; to bring in that additional oomph to the main act of lovemaking.

Many regions in a human body like the neck area, the thigh area, the inner calves, lower backs and the love handles are often neglected from the adoration and attention that they deserve. Many people mistake the love handles, which is the cute and trimmed layer of fat around your waist seen with scores of men and women, as unwanted flab.

But in reality, this region is laced with nerve endings and caressing it with accurate care can bring immense joy to your partner. Drawing parallel from that experience, love handles can be teased and squeezed to induce a feeling of delightful satisfaction in your heart.

Whether you are the receiving partner or the giving partner, you will thoroughly enjoy the synapses fired up and the responses developed from the sensual assault on your senses.

A lingering touch with your palms grazing over the lower back of your partner will not only tug at their ticklish ribs but also fire up their sexual glands and have them feeling racy and hot for the incoming pitch. To add to the bonus, it isn't very far off from the lower back to the upper backside and firm circular movements all over the backside can be very enticing to both the participants.

How would you let your partner know that you are enjoying the slow seduction of your senses? It is often essential to be communicative to enhance the development of eroticism in your relationship. A lingering squirm of your beautiful curvaceous butt against the throbbing mast can send hormones flying into a frenzy.

A soft wriggle of the waist can help magnify a sensual strip-show. Sneaking up on your partner and letting them have a whiff of your favourite cologne will leave them desiring for much more.

Use of choice objects to extract more pleasure out of an otherwise bland experience will shoot the erotic factor up and out of the roof. Ornamental objects like anal beads may not sound as appealing but the continual jiggle while enjoying moments of intimacy with your partner can onset some very arousing feelings.

Similarly, the gradual assault of a vibrator not just down the conventional road, but on and around offbeat body parts can send little shoots of joy down your spine.

One of the most important and significant elements of psychological love can be the skill of kissing romantically. Be it at the end of a date or at the beginning of a lovemaking session, a kiss holds prime importance. It has the decisive and the definitive power. A romantic and passionate kiss has the power of throwing you off balance and sending you into a spiraling cave of ecstasy more enjoyable than the ride down a water slide at an amusement park.

The French have discovered a very fool-proof way of perfecting the skill, the swift and jovial movements of the tongue in a flamboyant dance with your partner's can be deeply satisfying.

Lousy kisses filled with mundane traction are not likely to please your partner, or satisfy them in any way. You may even choose to suckle at your partner's bottom lip. Even benign efforts are sure to arouse your partner's subconscious and have them pumped up for much more.

The main target of learning the art of eroticism is to make yourself and your partner feel sexy. The accompaniment of such appetizers will make the meal seem all the more delicious and tantalizing.

And only the meals that completely satisfy you in every way possible are like to be savored again and again, not the bland ones that pitifully lack the burst of spices and fall short of your high expectations from a great looking package.

Conclusion

Thank you again for purchasing this book!

I hope this book has helped you understand that sex is beyond a list of how to please your partner to achieve orgasms. Sex is sacred in the true sense because it is a union of two bodies dissolving into one consciousness.

To experience healthy sex lives, couples need to take a look at what happened along the way. Familiarity breeds contempt, that's the order of things and so, is change, change is constant, and being able to see things from a non-judgmental perspective is the first step towards a healthy relationship.

Accept your partner as they are; address your concerns in a positive manner that helps them understand what's been bothering you. Nagging and blaming don't lead to solutions, instead they fan the sparks to conflict, and couples grow distant due to this nasty habit.

When issues among couples are resolved, sex life

improves. If at some point you feel the need to consult a therapist, do so as early as possible to gain back the life you fear might be slipping away.

Finally, if you enjoyed this book, then I'd like to ask you for a favor, would you be kind enough to leave a review for this book on Amazon? It'd be greatly appreciated!

Thank you and good luck!

Check Out My Other Books

Below you'll find some of my other popular books that are popular on Amazon and Kindle as well. Simply click on the links below to check them out.

Alternatively, you can visit my author page on Amazon to see other work done by me. You can type my name (Tracy Willowbank) into Amazon and you will also see new books I'm adding all the time.

Butt Workout
How To be Good At Sex

Do You Want More Books?

How would you like books arriving in your inbox each week?

They're FREE!

We publish books on all sorts of non-fiction niches and send them to our subscribers each week to spread the love.

All you have to do is sign up and you're good to go!

Just go to the link below, sign up, sit back and wait for your book downloads to arrive.

We couldn't have made it any easier. Enjoy!

www.LibraryBugs.com

Manufactured by Amazon.ca
Bolton, ON